Breakfast
is
*Bullsh*t*

I0505754

How You Will Lose Weight and
Become Healthier by Skipping the
Most Important Meal of the Day

by
K.D. Joseph

If you would like to contact the author with any questions please email:

kdjosephadvice@gmail.com

CONTENTS

CHAPTER 1

"The rest of the world lives to eat,
while I eat to live."
- Socrates

BREAKFAST is the most overrated meal of the day.

In this short book you will see that if you want to be healthier, and lose unwanted weight, you should stop eating breakfast. There is simply no need to be eating in the morning, and your body will be grateful if you give up this unnecessary dietary habit.

If the idea of skipping breakfast for health reasons seems shocking to you, it won't be once you are finished reading this guide. The popular opinion of breakfast being the most important meal of the day is a myth. And if you skip breakfast for yourself over the next few weeks you will get to pleasantly experience this fact for yourself.

Skipping breakfast has quietly become more accepted over the last few years in some nutrition circles, because it is one of the key components of the popular dietary movement known as intermittent fasting. However, too many books about intermittent fasting are unnecessarily confusing, longwinded, and often miss the bigger picture altogether.

This guide will be your antidote to that. It will also provide you with a few deeper insights into why we as a culture tend to overeat without even noticing it, and how you can easily stop doing this.

So relax and read the following pages knowing there's nothing special or complicated you need to memorize. What you're about to read is simple to understand, and there's never any pressure on you. When you're finished with the material, feel free to email me if you have any additional questions. I'm here to help if you need it. Once you feel relaxed, let's begin with a brief overview of why intermittent fasting has seen a surge in popularity…

Intermittent fasting, for the vast majority of people who safely want to lose weight, simply entails skipping breakfast and not eating anything after dinner. That's it.

This simple advice, which is diametrically opposed to most standard American dietary recommendations, can significantly improve your health. Intermittent fasting is easy, hence its growing popularity.

I personally have tried many dietary options in my life (vegetarian, raw food, low-carb, protein cycling – to name a few) and the intermittent fasting model is by far the easiest diet to implement and stay on that I have ever come across. The reasons for that are pretty self-explanatory.

Many diets claim to be simple, but end up being difficult. What's brilliant about intermittent fasting is that it backs up all its claims of being rather effortless. All you need to do is skip breakfast and stop eating food once dinner is over. This setup means you end up consuming all your calories for the day in a much shorter window of time than most people do.

For instance, you might eat lunch at noon, and then you'll be finished with dinner at 8pm. You didn't start eating until around lunchtime, and you stopped eating once dinner ended. All your calories were consumed in that eight hour span. Some days that eating window might be slightly shorter, and some days a little longer, but you get the gist. Your eating window should be between five to nine hours long on most days.

Intermittent fasting is manageable to start and sustain, because it's so blatantly simple to follow. You naturally consume fewer calories over the course of the day by not eating anything in the morning and late at night. And, inevitably, you lose weight because of this dietary habit.

Simple caloric restriction like this intuitively makes sense as a concept for weight loss, and it works. So just start trying it out. Begin skipping breakfast and don't eat until around lunchtime. For some people lunch means 11am, for others it means 2:30pm. Wait to eat lunch until you honestly feel hungry; feelings of hunger might come at slightly different times for you each day, and let this hunger be your guide as opposed to a set time on the clock.

In the morning you can still be drinking water. You can also drink tea or black coffee, because there are essentially no calories in those drinks. But don't consume any real calories until lunch. Once lunch begins, your "fast" is over and your eating window for the day has started. At night, once you have had dinner, don't snack on anything, and try not to drink alcohol after your meal (a tip for those who want to have a drink or two after dinner – don't start eating the next day until the mid-afternoon.) Your eating window is done for the day as soon as dinner has finished.

So relax, smile, and realize this is all you have to do to master the simple art of intermittent fasting:

Skip breakfast, and don't eat after dinner. That's it.

CHAPTER 2

*"We never regret of having
eaten too little."
- Thomas Jefferson*

OF course, intermittent fasting can be described much more elaborately, but for almost all of us, it just comes back to skipping breakfast and not eating late into the night. No need to make it more complicated. *You want to just try doing it, and see the pleasant results for yourself.*

Don't obsess over unnecessary details; just start skipping breakfast. This first simple step is the most important step by far. So let's spend a moment talking about the act of skipping breakfast. This is all you need to know:

It's not hard to skip breakfast.

Don't worry, you won't starve if you don't have your bagel in the morning. People eat much more often than they need to. We don't need to be eating every few hours. Nor is there the need to constantly be thinking about food. We mentally obsess over food when there's no reason to do so. Do you ever notice that when we're very busy and skip a meal, we don't notice our hunger until afterwards? That is because we weren't thinking about eating when we were busy. We aren't hungry unless we *think* we're hungry.

You don't have to eat more than two or three times a day – at most – and there's absolutely no point to eating in the morning. *We eat more often, and often much more, than we probably should.* We do this because we're mentally ingrained with the habit of eating a lot and eating often.

Here's the good news – it's not at all necessary to eat this way, and your body knows this. Actually, your body will be extremely pleased if you start eating less food, and less often. You'll know your body is grateful because you'll feel better, and you'll probably become leaner.

This has nothing to do with deprivation – I'm opposed to denying ourselves what we enjoy eating – and everything to do with switching our *mindset* towards eating and hunger.

CHAPTER 3

"You eat not food but ideas."
- U.G. Krishnamurti

I know skipping breakfast goes against what many nutritionists recommend, and that's okay. What some nutritionists think is right isn't always based upon actual reality. This health advice you're reading now is pragmatic and explicitly about reality. It's not theoretical or abstract. Thousands of years of human history – human reality – indicates that it's best not to be constantly eating, or to be overeating simply out of habit.

Eat less, feel better.

This has nothing to do with deprivation; it's an effortless act based upon a simple shift of consciousness. Don't deprive yourself of what you want when you're legitimately hungry. But also don't eat just for the heck of it. Eat when you're hungry. Otherwise, don't eat.

Don't be concerned about not having "energy" because you didn't eat in the morning, or because you have gone more than a few hours without a meal. Our hunter-gatherer ancestors regularly went *days* without eating – and they were probably healthier than most of us. This is not a coincidence. Those feelings of low energy from not eating every few hours are purely psychological.

Any initial feelings of fatigue you experience when you start skipping breakfast will go away after a couple of days, and are mainly a small mental hurdle you need to overcome. Let me reassure you that such feelings of physical weakness are almost always strictly mental. We *think* we're weak from not eating, but we're actually no weaker. Don't worry, after a few days our slightly neurotic thoughts about morning hunger will disappear. They have no validity.

Eat a satisfying meal for dinner, and don't worry about eating until the following day at lunch. After only a few days of practice, this eating arrangement will seem normal.

There's no problem feeling a little hungry for lunch, whether that's around noon or a few hours later. Feeling a little bit of hunger is good; it's a natural part of our biological process. Often many of us aren't hungry when we wake up, but we're accustomed to having breakfast because we're "supposed to." We're slaves to this mental habit, and it's time to free ourselves of this burden.

Let me repeat myself for the sake of clarity. You can still drink liquid – like water, black coffee or tea – but consume no calories before lunch. For the first couple of days this might be mildly difficult, but gently battle through it. It's not hard. Relax and understand that soon you'll be mentally used to not eating in the morning, and it will actually be enjoyable to never worry about what you need to eat for breakfast.

If you can hold off eating until lunch, and presuming you haven't eaten since dinner the night before, then each day you're giving your body a long window in which you're not consuming any calories. Performing this simple act is incredibly advantageous to weight loss, and also helpful to your general health.

When we do sit down and eat, we should eat until we feel full. We should try our best to eat slowly, chew our food and not needlessly overeat – but we absolutely should not be "watching" our calories. We should simply eat until we feel satiated, and then stop. If we do this, there's no need to be eating every few hours, or to be snacking constantly.

Try having only two or three meals a day, and cut out the pattern of eating all the time. Don't incessantly be nibbling on something. At noon you can have a big lunch, if you feel you need it. If you get hungry in the mid-afternoon, you can have a snack if you feel you need it (the blunt truth is we almost always snack out of habit, not out of necessity. That's not pointing fingers; it's just the truth.) You can have a big dinner at night, if you need it. That will be plenty of food for the day – you'll be full, believe me.

Ideally your dinner will be on the early side, instead of later at night. It's probably better to be done consuming calories at 7pm as opposed to 10pm, but regardless of when you stop eating in the evening, all of your caloric consumption is confined to a somewhat limited window of time. This makes a big difference, and is why this eating model works so well for all types of people.

CHAPTER 4

"If you are to live according to the 'Science of Being Well,' you must never eat until you have an earned hunger. But if I do not eat on arising in the morning, when shall I take my first meal? In 99 cases out of 100, twelve o'clock noon is early enough, and it is generally the most convenient time. If you are doing heavy work, you will get by noon a hunger sufficient to justify a good-sized meal. And if your work is light, you will probably still have hunger enough for a moderate meal. The best general rule or law that can be laid down is that you should eat your first meal of the day at noon if you are hungry, and if you are not hungry, wait until you become so."

- Wallace Wattles

IT'S not required that you follow this eating pattern and skip breakfast every day, *but it's very strongly recommended.* It's so easy for us not to eat until lunchtime.

Once you overcome the small mental hurdles of the first few days your body and mind simply get used to not eating until around lunchtime. From there it's smooth sailing. You still might feel some very minor hunger pangs as lunch approaches, but nothing more. Wait to eat until your body honestly tells you it's ready. Then your lunch, whatever it is, will be satisfying.

And please don't believe you "need" to have breakfast. This stand-ard dietary suggestion is grounded in no truth whatsoever. The assertion that we need to have a healthy breakfast to have a healthy lifestyle is absurd, particularly if we're inter-ested in losing weight. Think about it. Instead of having a meal at seven or eight o'clock in the morning, we hold off until lunch-time. That extra four or five hours without food is significant.

If you still think skipping breakfast won't work for you, at least cut down on how much you eat in the morning. For instance, you could have a cup of coffee with heavy cream. That's pretty filling. But you don't need to eat a big breakfast. If you really like breakfast, have it for lunch – have bacon and eggs with coffee at 1pm instead of at 8am.

If your schedule makes it easier to skip dinner and only have breakfast and lunch every day, that setup works too. You will still have that advantageously smaller eating window. The same model applies whether you skip breakfast or dinner.

That's the entire eating formula in a nutshell, and all the info that most of us will ever want to know on the subject. If there is one thing I need to emphasize, it is this:

This is easy.

Don't make these simple eating tips hard for yourself; it should all be easy. Just relax, you'll get it right. Don't worry about being perfect; just try your best and everything will quickly fall into place.

Other easy tips to rapidly improve your health include getting ample sleep and taking a large Vitamin D3 supplement daily along with a Vitamin K2 supplement. Vitamin D3 and Vitamin K2 work strangely well together in promoting good health.

These simple health recommendations are all basic enough that you can start doing them immediately without difficulty, and they work very well – which is the only thing that's truly important.

CHAPTER 5

"I saw few die of hunger;
of eating, a hundred thousand."
- Benjamin Franklin

NOT to be overly repetitive, but let me mention this again: please don't worry about being hungry.

People get worried that they'll be detrimentally hungry if they start skipping breakfast, as if the lack of food in the morning will destroy their lives. After a few days of actually skipping breakfast, you'll realize how ridiculous a fear this is.

The truth is that in our modern culture, the vast majority of people overeat. Hunger is a mental thing, not a physical thing. Our human body is pretty incredible. Even as amazing as modern medicine is, our body is still usually its own best healer. But our body works best when we generally leave it alone and don't constantly overfeed it.

Hunger is mental in our culture.

It's worth remembering that. Be gentle and loving of your body, and try not to overeat. Then watch your health naturally improve without effort, simply by not interfering with your body's incredible, inherent healing powers. Assume health, and become healthy. If you follow these simple steps, and begin to feel yourself as already being healthy, then health will follow.

Not eating until you are truly hungry is a rather intuitive thing, when we're not unnecessarily neurotic about eating and food (all of us, unfortunately, can think of times when we have been neurotic about what we eat.) Skipping breakfast allows you the pleasure of not overeating, not overanalyzing what you eat, and a better enjoyment of whatever you do decide to eat.

Take advantage of this wonderfully simple eating model, there's little reason not to. The most important thing is not when you eat, but not overeating simply for the sake of it. Take breakfast, excess food consumption, and constantly worrying about your body out of the equation. You deserve better than that, and you'll be amazed how much better you feel when you begin doing it.

Start enjoying eating in a more meaningful way. If you can give this gift to yourself, your body will gratefully thank you, and you'll be rewarded with better health, naturally.

CHAPTER 6

"Let your food be your medicine
and your medicine be your food."
- Hippocrates

ONCE you understand the psychological component of hunger, everything changes. Your body usually
performs better when it takes in less
food, less often. To do this we do not
try to deprive ourselves of what we
like eating – because such deprivation usually does not work – but
instead simply shift our attitude and
mindset towards hunger.

To further clarify this point, if you
are interested, let me now provide
some quotes from two masters on the
subject. You don't have to read these
quotes to start skipping breakfast
and see the pleasant results. Consider this simply a bonus section to
the guide, and one you might enjoy.

Wallace Wattles is the author of the
self-help classic *"The Science of Being
Well."* This book is over a hundred
years old, and although parts of it
seem outdated, it still blows most

modern health books away. Here's a nice tidbit from it —

Appetite is often largely a matter of habit; if one eats or drinks at a certain hour, and especially if one takes sweetened or spiced and stimulating foods, the desire comes regularly at the same hour; but this habitual desire for food should never be mistaken for hunger. Hunger does not appear at specified times. It only comes when work or exercise has destroyed sufficient tissue to make the taking in of new raw material a necessity.

For instance, if a person has been sufficiently fed on the preceding day, it is impossible that he should feel a genuine hunger on arising from refreshing sleep. In sleep the body is recharged with vital power, and the assimilation of the food which has been taken during the day is completed; the system has no need for food immediately after sleep, unless the person went to his rest in a state of starvation. With a system of feeding, which is even a reasonable approach to a natural one, no one can have a real hunger for an early morning breakfast. There is no such thing possible as a normal or genuine hunger immediately after arising from sound sleep. The early morning breakfast is always taken to gratify appetite, never to satisfy hunger. No matter who you are, or what your condition is; no matter how hard you work, or how much you are exposed, unless you go to your bed starved, you cannot arise from your bed hungry.

Hunger is not caused by sleep, but by work. And it does not matter who you are, or what your condition, or how hard or easy your work, the so-called no-breakfast plan is the right plan for you. It is the right plan for everybody, because it is based on the universal law that hunger never comes until it is EARNED.

I am aware that a protest against this will come from the large number of people who "enjoy" their breakfasts; whose breakfast is their "best meal;" who believe that their work is so hard that they cannot "get through the forenoon on an empty stomach," and so on. But all their arguments fall down before the facts. They enjoy their breakfast as the toper enjoys his morning dram, because it gratifies a habitual appetite and not because it supplies a natural want. It is their best meal for the same reason that his morning dram is the toper's best drink. And they CAN get along without it, because millions of people, of every trade and profession, DO get along without it, and are vastly better for doing so. If you are to live according to the Science of Being Well, you must NEVER EAT UNTIL YOU HAVE AN EARNED HUNGER.

But if I do not eat on arising in the morning, when shall I take my first meal?

In 99 cases out of a 100 twelve o'clock, noon, is early enough; and it is generally the most convenient time. If you are doing heavy work, you will get by noon a hunger sufficient to justify a good-sized meal; and if your work is light, you will probably still have hunger enough for a moderate meal. The best general rule or law that can be laid down is that you should eat your first meal of the day at noon, if you are hungry; and if you are not hungry, wait until you become so.

And when shall I eat my second meal?

Not at all, unless you are hungry for it; and that with a genuine earned hunger. If you do get hungry for a second meal, eat at the most convenient time; but do not eat until you have a really earned hunger.

Wattles' book is a worthwhile read, if you are curious.

Another master at understanding the subject of overeating, if you really want to delve deeper into it, was the brilliantly iconoclastic philosopher U.G. Krishnamurti (everybody just called him U.G.) He believed we ate excessively based out of cultural habit, and that our body naturally functions *much better and more peacefully* when we do not constantly try to interfere with it.

U.G. lived to be 88 years old without seeking medical help the last half century of his life. He was unusually alive and energetic for a person of any age, traveling extensively well into his eighties. U.G. ate very little, and he would eat whatever he wanted. Here are a few disarming quotes from U.G. about food and the human body —

The body needs some energy, and that energy you can have from anything you eat. Sawdust is enough for it, without the health food and vitamin C, or your brown rice and seaweed.

You can believe whatever you want to believe. Someone else believes something else. It is the belief that matters to people. You replace one belief with another. You eat ideas. You put ideas in your stomach. You can eat good ideas. Good luck to you.

The moment you ask, "How to live?" and "What to eat?" you have created a problem – everything is cultural. All your tastes are cultivated tastes. The body does not know what you are eating. The problem is you eat more than what the body needs. It's the overeating that is the problem. You eat for pleasure. Eating has become a pleasure seeking movement for us.

The body needs food. The moment you introduce the question of "right" food you have introduced control there. The stomach can digest anything, but we put ideas into the stomach, and the capacity, the micro-function of the stomach, is destroyed.

—————————————

You see, if it were possible for you to eat – it doesn't matter what it is, whether it is pasta or whatever it is – if you can eat without this thought structure operating, then you are eating. Instead, what you do is this: the moment you eat something you begin to recognize the taste – it is salty or it is sweet. But without this process all the time functioning inside of you, you will feel extraordinarily peaceful.

This is because of a physical action. The blood rushes to the stomach because the stomach needs the blood. If I am thinking while I am eating, I am thinking because I recognize the taste, I remember my likes and dislikes – all this thinking process is continuing. I am thinking and eating at the same time. That is why some religious orders prohibit you from talking. That doesn't help because even if I am not talking, I am thinking inside. All the time the thoughts are going on. So there is no enjoyment there.

So, if one can eat without thinking, the blood rushes to the stomach. The stomach needs the blood when you eat something. The rushing of the blood to the stomach produces an extraordinary peace that passes understanding. There is an enjoyment – pure enjoyment. But in your case what is going on is pleasure. Pleasure is a repetitive process. I am not saying anything against pleasure. But it is a repetitive process, and so it is wearing out the senses.

I am talking about pure and simple living with your senses to the fullest possible extent. What I am trying to do is put you in a state of non-awareness. This exploration takes place if it is a totally different way of living with your senses. That means you let these senses operate in their own way. It is not a mystical thing. It has nothing to do with mysticism at all. This is a pure and simple functioning of the senses to the fullest possible extent.

This human body is not interested in learning or knowing anything. All that is necessary for the survival of this living organism is already there. There is a tremendous intelligence there, and all that we have gathered and acquired through our intellect is no match for that.

The first time when you eat something, maybe you enjoy it. The second time, you are not enjoying anything at all. There is no enjoyment. We are not enjoying at all – we are living in the world of pleasure. Pleasure means repetition. I want exactly the way the sweets have tasted before. So I am eating my memories – I am not eating the thing that is there.

Whatever is there in the body is there in the body to use. There is a surplus energy for you to do whatever you want to do. It is there all the time.

This body is born with an extraordinary intelligence, unparalleled intelligence. And there is no way you can match this with any amount of knowledge you have. You cannot. So, whatever you think is good for this body, whatever ideas you are putting into this body, it is rejecting. That is why it doesn't need to know anything, it doesn't need to have anything more. That applies to every area of our existence. That's why I brush aside the whole medical technology. I have never been to a doctor, I don't eat anything that anybody recommends and I say emphatically that modern day doctors are the modern day witches, and modern day medical technology is the modern day witchcraft, as far as I am concerned. Whatever they think is good for the body, I don't eat.

I eat that oatmeal there. That is the latest I find, it's called "Super Fast."

You can find it only in London. I have one bowl, a small bowl and then pour double cream, triple cream, quadruple cream and I add a tiny weenie bit of frozen pineapple juice, which I don't get anywhere except in China. That's why I go to China. They have international supermarkets. So, otherwise I don't take fruit juices, I don't eat any vegetables. Nothing. You see, this body needs some energy, some basic thermal units. You see, that's how I would put it. And that one bowl of oatmeal porridge with a lot of cream, supplies the energy that the body needs. I don't take walks and no exercise is necessary. I have survived eighty years. So nothing of what we consider to be good for the body is actually good for this body.

So, what I am stressing all the time is how the body, freed from this stranglehold of culture, functions. That's all that I am describing. And there is no way you can control the functioning of this body. Nothing you can do, you see. The body doesn't actually need all that we feed it. It is a pleasure movement. We eat for our pleasure. That's a fact.

Surely you eat things for your pleasure and not for your body. We develop a habit. If you watch for yourself you'll know. If you deny some food you like you'll see how the mind is working. Sitting at the dining table is the thing. The recognition of food, its taste – all of them are interrelated. When you are eating you are thinking and you are destroying the full possibility of what the food can give you. This thinking process needs blood in the brain which actually is needed in the stomach. That is why there is a traditional saying that you should not talk nor think while eating.

Here, what happens is that when I eat – since I'm not thinking and I don't even know what I'm eating, its taste and all that – the food goes to the stomach and immediately there is a rush of blood to the stomach and that produces great bliss. This bliss is not the result of meditation or something; it is there because the blood has gone where it is necessary. This is the natural function-ing of the body.

The body has intelligence of its own. Give it a chance. The human intellect we have cultivated over millions of years is no match to this intelligence of the body. It'll take care of itself. So you can't eat wrong food.

If you want more from U.G. there is a great free "cookbook" by Julie Thayer that cuts to the essence of what U.G is talking about. It's not really the recipes in the cookbook that are important, but U.G.'s insightful philosophy concerning eating. You will find the cookbook online if you do a search for it.

After reading Wattles and U.G.'s thoughts on food, you will never be worried about missing breakfast again. But this goes way beyond just skipping breakfast. We mainly eat out of pleasure, not necessity. If we recognize this fact, something powerful shifts in terms of how we eat, and we naturally become healthier. Hopefully this guide has helped you recognize this plain truth. Naturally eating less is easy, and it works wonders for our health.

If you have questions regarding this material, or any general questions, feel free to email me at:

kdjosephadvice@gmail.com

Thanks for reading, and cheers to your health!

- K.D.

*Another simple guide by
K.D. Joseph you might enjoy:*

The 5-Second Cure

*Your Surprisingly Simple
Solution to Avoid Getting Sick
and Beat Disease Naturally*

This short guide is going to show you a simple, uniquely effective way to avoid getting sick. It will help you substantially reduce the number of common colds and cases of the flu you get for the rest of your life.

In short, if you hate getting sick, you should read these suggestions.

The bonus of this guide, for the curious reader, is that it can also show you how to treat and cure more serious health problems in an easier way. The essence of this material contains deeper implications than just learning how to treat the common cold.

www.ingramcontent.com/pod-product-compliance
Lightning Source LLC
Chambersburg PA
CBHW071001180526
45168CB00003B/1242